THE 7-DAY DASH DIET MEAL PLAN

The Ultimate Program to Lose Weight, Lower Blood Pressure, and Prevent Diabetes

Rosemary Anderson

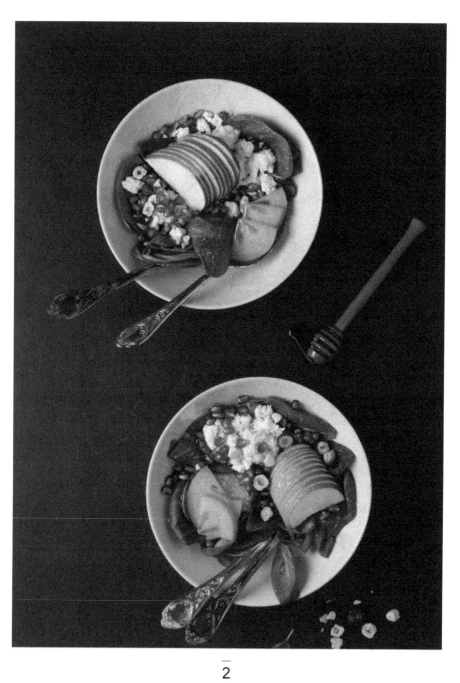

TABLE OF CONTENTS

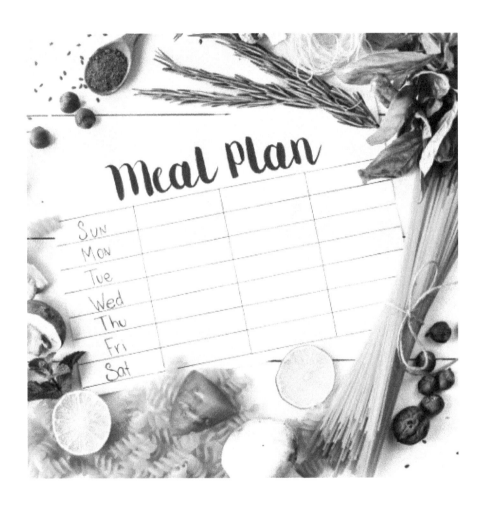

Meal Plan

Sun			
Mon			
Tue			
Wed			
Thu			
Fri			
Sat			

DAY 1

BREAKFAST: Apple-Cinnamon Baked Oatmeal

SNACK A.M.: 6 oz. light yogurt, nonfat

1½ oz. almonds

LUNCH: Minty Chickpea Tabbouleh

Snack P.M.: 1 medium pear, sliced topped with cinnamon

DINNER: Pasta with Grilled Chicken

NUTRITIONAL VALUES:

Kcal: 1333

Sodium: 528 mg

Protein: 41 g

Carbs: 134 g

Fat: 22 g

TO MAKE IT 1500 KCAL ADD:

¼ cup unsalted dry-roasted almonds to breakfast

1 medium banana to lunch

TO MAKE IT 2000 KCAL ADD:

¼ cup unsalted dry-roasted almonds to breakfast

¼ cup walnuts to A.M. snack

1 banana and a 1 oz. slice of whole-wheat baguette to lunch

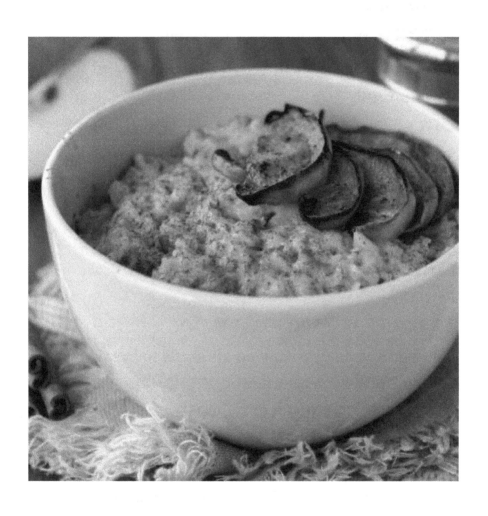

Apple-Cinnamon Baked Oatmeal

🕐 **Ready in about: 50 min**

🍴 **Serves: 8**

🍎 **Per serving: Kcal 312, Sodium 4 mg, Protein 9 g, Carbs 60 g, Fat 7.5 g**

INGREDIENTS

- **2 cups steel-cut oats**
- **8 cups of water**
- **1 tsp. cinnamon**
- **½ tsp. allspice**
- **½ tsp. nutmeg**
- **¼ cup brown sugar**
- **1 tsp. vanilla extract**
- **2 apples, diced**
- **1 cup raisins**

- ½ cup unsalted, roasted walnuts, chopped

DIRECTIONS

1. Spray the cooker with non-stick cooking spray.
2. Add all the ingredients to the cooker except the nuts.
3. Mix well to combine. Put the cooker on low heat for 30 minutes.
4. Serve garnished with chopped walnuts.

Minty Chickpea Tabbouleh

🕐 **Ready in about: 30 min**

🍴 **Serves: 4**

🍎 **Per serving: Kcal 380, Sodium 450 mg, Protein 4 g, Carbs 21 g, Fat 3 g**

INGREDIENTS

- ½ tsp. salt
- ¼ tsp. pepper
- 2 tbsp. lemon juice
- ¼ cup olive oil
- 2 tbsp. julienned soft sun-dried tomatoes
- ¼ cup minced fresh mint
- 1 can (15 oz.) of garbanzo beans or chickpeas (rinsed and drained)
- ½ cup minced fresh parsley
- 1 cup fresh or frozen peas (thawed)

13

- 1 cup bulgur
- 2 cups water

DIRECTIONS

1. Put water and bulgur in a pan over medium-high flame and bring to a boil.

2. Turn heat to low, cover the pan and simmer for 10 minutes.

3. Add peas, stir and cover the pan.

4. Lower the pressure of the heat and simmer for 5 minutes or until the peas and bulgur are cooked.

5. Put the cooked dish in a bowl and add the rest of the ingredients.

6. Serve warm.

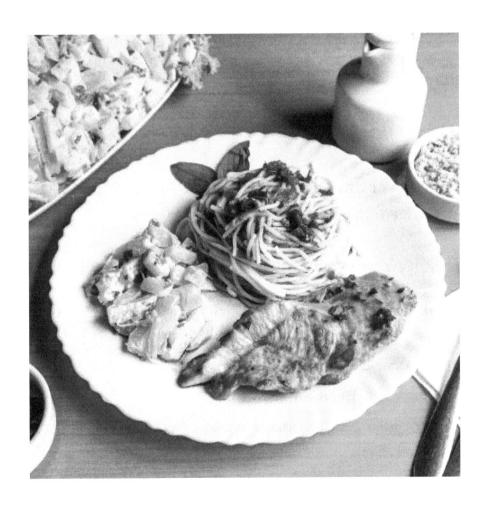

Pasta with Grilled Chicken

🕐 **Ready in about: 45 min**

🍴 **Serves: 6**

🍎 **Per serving: Kcal 341, Sodium 74 mg, Protein 21 g, Carbs 53.5 g, Fat 5 g**

INGREDIENTS

- 2 boneless, skinless chicken breasts, each 4 oz.
- 1 tbsp. olive oil
- ½ cup chopped white onion
- 1 cup sliced mushrooms
- 1 cup white beans, canned or cooked (no salt added)
- 2 tbsp. chopped garlic
- ¼ cup chopped fresh basil
- 12 oz. uncooked rotelle pasta
- ¼ cup grated Parmesan cheese

- Ground black pepper, to taste

DIRECTIONS

1. In a coal grill, prepare a hot fire or heat up a broiler or gas grill.

2. Away from sources of heat, coat grill or pan lightly with cooking spray.

3. Place the cooking rack 4 to 6 inches from the heat source.

4. Broil or grill the chicken until golden brown and just cooked through, about 5 minutes per side.

5. Shift the chicken to a cutting board before cutting into strips and let it rest for 5 minutes.

6. In an enormous nonstick skillet, heat olive oil over medium heat.

7. Add onions and mushrooms and sauté until tender, about 5 minutes.

8. Add the white beans, garlic, basil and grilled chicken strips. Keep warm.

9. Fill ¾ of a large saucepan with water and bring it to a boil.

10. Add the pasta and cook until tender, for 10 to 12 minutes or as directed by the packet.

11. Drain the pasta well. Return the pasta to the pot and add the chicken mixture.

12. Stir to mix evenly. Divide the pasta between the plates.

13. Garnish each with 1 tbsp. of Parmesan and black pepper. Serve immediately.

DAY 2

BREAKFAST: Healthy French Toast

SNACK A.M.: 1 medium banana

LUNCH: Cream of Wild Rice Hot Dish & Apple-Fennel Slaw

Snack P.M.: Fruit and Nut Bar

DINNER: Basil Halibut

NUTRITIONAL VALUES:

Kcal: 1212

Sodium: 802 mg

Protein: 64 g

Carbs: 90.5 g

Fat: 60 g

TO MAKE IT 1500 KCAL. ADD:

¼ cup walnut halves to breakfast

1 medium pear to lunch

TO MAKE IT 2000 KCAL. ADD:

¼ cup walnut halves to breakfast

1 medium pear to lunch

2 cups mixed greens and ½ avocado to dinner

Healthy French Toast

🕐 Ready in about: 15 min.

🍴 Serves: 4

🍎 Per serving: Kcal 305, Sodium 438 mg, Protein 15 g, Carbs 49 g, Fat 7 g

INGREDIENTS

- 4 egg whites
- 1 whole egg
- 1 cup unsweetened almond milk
- ½ tsp. ground cinnamon
- 1 tsp. vanilla extract
- ¼ tsp. ground nutmeg
- ½ tsp. powdered stevia
- 8 slices whole-grain bread (at least ½-1 inch thick)

DIRECTIONS

1. Combine the egg whites, whole egg, almond milk, cinnamon, vanilla, nutmeg and stevia in a shallow bowl.

2. Plunge each slice of bread in the mixture for about 1 minute per side so that the bread absorbs the liquid and aromas.

3. Heat a grill pan until very hot and coat it with olive oil.

4. Place each soaked slice of bread on the griddle and bake for about 3 minutes per side, or until golden brown and crisp.

5. Serve immediately.

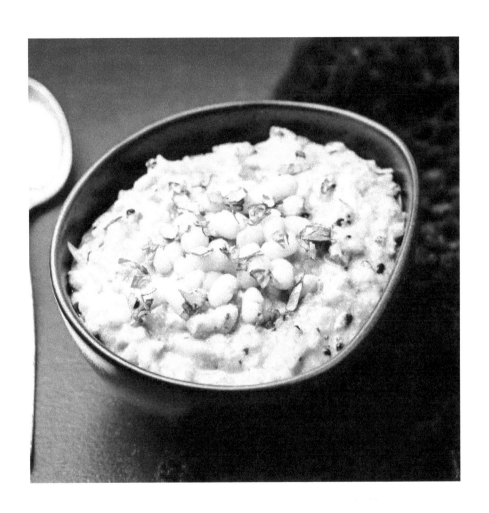

Cream of Wild Rice Hot Dish

🕐 **Ready in about: 50 min.**

🍴 **Serves: 4**

🍎 **Per serving: Kcal 236, Sodium 180 mg, Protein 25 g, Carbs 19 g, Fat 25 g**

INGREDIENTS

- 1 cup diced celery
- 2 cloves garlic, minced
- 1 cup diced carrot
- ½ tbsp. canola oil
- 1½ cups diced yellow onion
- 1 tsp. fennel seeds, crushed
- 1 tbsp. minced parsley
- 2 cups low-sodium vegetable stock
- 1½ cups chopped kale
- 1 cup unsalted prepared white beans

- 1 tsp. ground black pepper
- ½ cup wild rice, cooked
- 2 cups 1 percent milk

DIRECTIONS

1. Warmth the oil in a soup pot over medium flame.
2. Add garlic, celery, carrot, and onion.
3. Cook until browned while constantly stirring.
4. Add spices, stock, parsley, and kale.
5. Stir and bring to a boil.
6. Put milk and beans in a food processor.
7. Process until pureed. Transfer to a pot with soup. Add rice and simmer for half an hour.

Apple-Fennel Slaw

🕐 **Ready in about: 25 min.**

🍴 **Serves: 4**

🍎 **Per serving: Kcal 124, Sodium 61 mg, Protein 2 g, Carbs 22 g, Fat 1 g**

INGREDIENTS

- 1 medium-sized fennel bulb, thinly sliced
- 1 large Granny Smith apple, cored and thinly sliced
- 2 carrots, grated
- 2 tbsp. raisins
- 1 tbsp. olive oil
- 1 tsp. sugar
- ½ cup apple juice
- 2 tbsp. apple cider vinegar
- 4 lettuce leaves

DIRECTIONS

1. In an enormous bowl, combine the fennel, apple, carrots and raisins to make the slaw.

2. Drizzle with olive oil, cover and refrigerate while you prepare the rest of the ingredients.

3. In a saucepan, combine the sugar and apple juice.

4. Put on medium heat and cook until reduced to about ¼ cup, about 10 minutes.

5. Remove from heat and let cool.

6. Include the apple cider vinegar.

7. Pour the apple juice mixture over the slaw and mix well.

8. Let cool completely.

9. Serve on lettuce leaves.

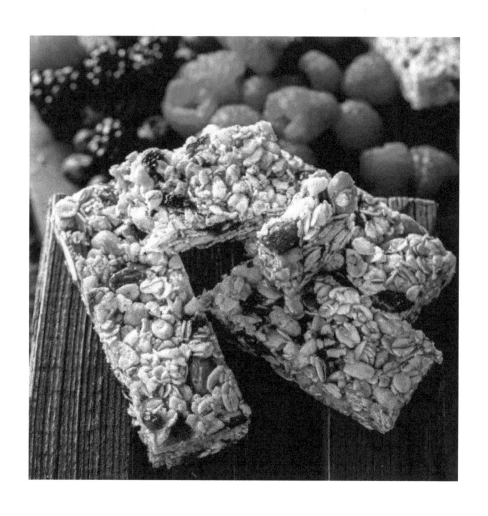

Fruit and Nut Bar

⏰ **Ready in about: 50 min.**

🍴 **Serves: 24**

🍎 **Per serving: Kcal 70, Sodium 4 mg, Protein 2 g, Carbs 11 g, Fat 2 g**

INGREDIENTS

- ½ cup oats
- ½ cup quinoa flour
- ¼ cup flaxseed flour
- ¼ cup chopped almonds
- ¼ cup wheat germ
- ¼ cup chopped dried apricots
- 2 tbsp. cornstarch
- ¼ cup honey

- ¼ cup chopped dried figs ¼ cup chopped dried pineapple

DIRECTIONS

1. Line a baking sheet with parchment paper.

2. Combine all the ingredients, mix well.

3. Press the mixture into the skillet until it is ½ inch thick.

4. Bake at 300°F for 20 minutes.

5. Let it cool completely and cut into 24 pieces.

Basil Halibut

🕐 **Ready in about: 20 min.**

🍴 **Serves: 4**

🍎 **Per serving: Kcal 347, Sodium 123 mg, Protein 22 g, Carbs 0.5 g, Fat 28 g**

INGREDIENTS

- **1-pound halibut, chopped**
- **1 tbsp. dried basil**
- **1 tsp. garlic powder**
- **2 tbsp. olive oil**

DIRECTIONS

1. Spurt the olive oil into the pan and heat it.

2. Meanwhile, combine halibut, dried basil and garlic powder.

3. Put the fish in the hot oil and coot it for 3 minutes on each side.

4. Dry oil and serve.

DAY 3

BREAKFAST: Chocolate Smoothie

SNACK A.M.: 6 oz. strawberries

LUNCH: Sweet Potato Balls

Snack P.M.: 5 dried figs

DINNER: Turkey Soup

NUTRITIONAL VALUES:

Kcal: 1289

Sodium: 307 mg

Protein: 87 g

Carbs: 79 g

Fat: 46 g

TO MAKE IT 1500 KCAL. ADD:

¼ cup unsalted dry-roasted almonds to breakfast

1 medium apple to lunch

TO MAKE IT 2000 KCAL. ADD:

¼ cup unsalted dry-roasted almonds and 1 cup raspberries to breakfast

¼ cup walnuts to A.M. snack

1 apple and a 1 oz. slice of whole-wheat baguette to lunch

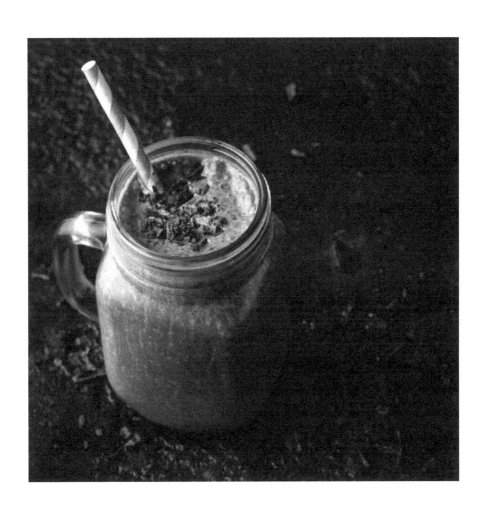

Chocolate Smoothie

🕐 Ready in about: 5 min.

🍴 Serves: 2

🍎 Per serving: Kcal 250, Sodium 134 mg, Protein 13 g, Carbs 31 g, Fat 11 g

INGREDIENTS

- 1 ripe banana, frozen at least overnight
- 2/3 cup low-fat (1%) milk
- 2/3 cup plain low-fat yogurt
- 2 tbsp. chunky peanut butter
- 2 tbsp. unsweetened cocoa powder
- 1 tbsp. amber agave nectar (optional)
- 4 ice cubes

DIRECTIONS

1. Peel and cut the banana into pieces.

2. In a blender, combine the banana with the milk, yogurt, peanut butter, cocoa powder, sweetener (if using) and ice cubes.

3. Pour into two tall glasses and serve immediately.

Sweet Potato Balls

🕐 **Ready in about: 25 min.**

🍴 **Serves: 2**

🍎 **Per serving: Kcal 122, Sodium 4 mg, Protein 8 g, Carbs 21 g, Fat 10.5 g**

INGREDIENTS

- 1 cup sweet potato, mashed, cooked
- 1 tbsp. fresh cilantro, chopped
- 1 egg, beaten
- 3 tbsp. ground oatmeal
- 1 tsp. ground paprika
- ½ tsp. ground turmeric
- 2 tbsp. coconut oil

DIRECTIONS

1. In the bowl, combine the mashed sweet potatoes, fresh cilantro, eggs, ground oatmeal, paprika, and turmeric.

2. Blend the mixture until smooth and make the small balls.

3. Heat the coconut oil in the pan.

4. Add the sweet potato balls to the hot coconut oil.

5. Cook them until golden brown.

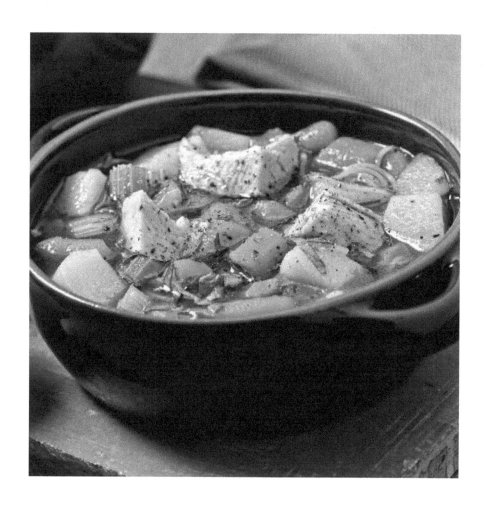

Turkey Soup

🕐 **Ready in about: 35 min.**

🍴 **Serves: 3**

🍎 **Per serving: Kcal 187, Sodium 131 mg, Protein 14 g, Carbs 17 g, Fat 8 g**

INGREDIENTS

- 1 potato, diced
- 1 cup ground turkey
- 1 tsp. cayenne pepper
- 1 onion, diced
- 1 tbsp. olive oil
- ¼ carrot, diced
- 2 cups of water

DIRECTIONS

1. Heat the olive oil in the pan and add the chopped onion and carrot.

2. Cook the vegetables for 3 minutes.

3. Mix well and add the ground turkey and cayenne pepper.

4. Add the chopped potato and mix the ingredients well.

5. Cook them for another 2 minutes. Then add the water.

6. Check if you put all the ingredients.

7. Cover and cook the soup for approximately 20 minute and serve hot.

DAY 4

BREAKFAST: Mediterranean Scramble

SNACK A.M.: 1 medium pear

LUNCH: Dash Diet Apple Sauce French Toast (2 servings)

Snack P.M.: 1 cup grapes

DINNER: Tofu Stroganoff & Spinach Berry Salad

NUTRITIONAL VALUES:

Kcal: 1256

Sodium: 1019 mg

Protein: 58 g

Carbs: 98 g

Fat: 61 g

TO MAKE IT 1500 KCAL. ADD:

¼ cup unsalted dry-roasted almonds to breakfast

1 small apple to lunch

TO MAKE IT 2000 KCAL. ADD:

¼ cup unsalted dry-roasted almonds and 1 cup raspberries to breakfast

¼ cup walnuts to A.M. snack

1 small apple to lunch

5 dried figs to P.M. snack

Mediterranean Scramble

🕐 **Ready in about: 15 min.**

🍴 **Serves: 1**

🍎 **Per serving: Kcal 424, Sodium 572 mg, Protein 21 g, Carbs 5 g, Fat 37 g**

INGREDIENTS

- 2 tbsp. extra virgin olive oil
- ⅛ cup chopped red onion
- 1 medium clove garlic, minced
- ¼ cup sliced red bell pepper
- ¼ cup rinsed and drained, chopped canned artichoke hearts
- 2 egg whites
- 1 whole egg
- ⅛ tsp. dried oregano
- ⅛ tsp. cracked black pepper

- ⅛ cup low-fat feta cheese

DIRECTIONS

1. Warmth a small non-stick pan over medium heat.

2. Add the oil to the hot pan, and when the oil is hot, add the onion and garlic.

3. Cook for 1 minute before adding the pepper strips and artichoke hearts.

4. Sauté vegetables for another 3 minutes or until onion is translucent and pepper is tender.

5. In a small bowl, beat the whites and egg until stiff and season with oregano and black pepper.

6. Pour in the eggs and mix them with a spatula.

7. Cook, 3 to 4 minutes or until the eggs are no longer runny.

8. Remove from heat, top with feta cheese and cover until the feta cheese begins to melt.

9. Serve immediately.

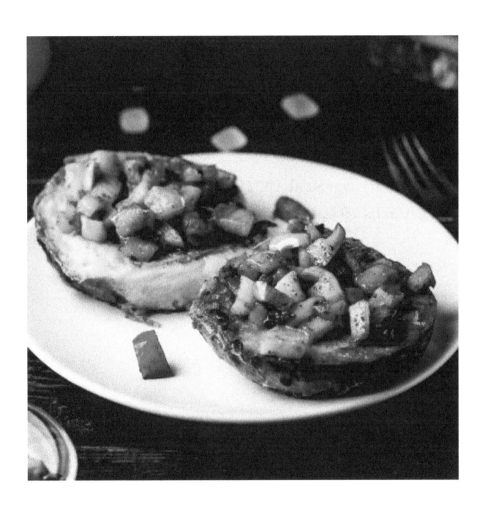

Dash Diet Apple Sauce French Toast

🕐 **Ready in about: 20 min.**

🍴 **Serves: 6**

🍎 **Per serving: Kcal 127, Sodium 206 mg, Protein 5.5 g, Carbs 19 g, Fat 3.5 g**

INGREDIENTS

- ¾ cup milk
- 2 eggs
- 6 slices bread
- 1 tsp. ground cinnamon
- ¼ cup applesauce
- 2 tbsp. white sugar

DIRECTIONS

1. In an enormous bowl, combine the eggs, milk, cinnamon, sugar, and applesauce; mix well.

2. Steep the bread one slice at a time until it is saturated with liquid.

3. Prepare in a lightly greased skillet or griddle over medium / high heat until lightly browned on both sides.

4. Serve hot.

Tofu Stroganoff

🕐 **Ready in about: 40 min.**

🍴 **Serves: 2**

🍎 **Per serving: Kcal 270, Sodium 49 mg, Protein 13 g, Carbs 28.5 g, Fat 12 g**

INGREDIENTS

- **4 oz. egg noodles**
- **6 oz. firm tofu, chopped**
- **1 tbsp. whole-wheat flour**
- **1 onion, sliced**
- **1 tbsp. coconut oil**
- **1 tsp. ground black pepper**
- **½ tsp. smoked paprika**
- **½ cup of soy milk**
- **½ cup of water**

DIRECTIONS

1. Grill the chopped onion with the coconut oil in the pan until golden brown.

2. Then add the ground black pepper, smoked paprika, water, and egg paste.

3. Boil the mixture for 8 minutes.

4. Then mix the flour and soy milk and pour the liquid into the stroganoff mixture.

5. Add the tofu and mix the mixture well.

6. Close the lid and cook the tofu stroganoff for 5 minutes.

7. Let the cooked food rest for 10 minutes and serve.

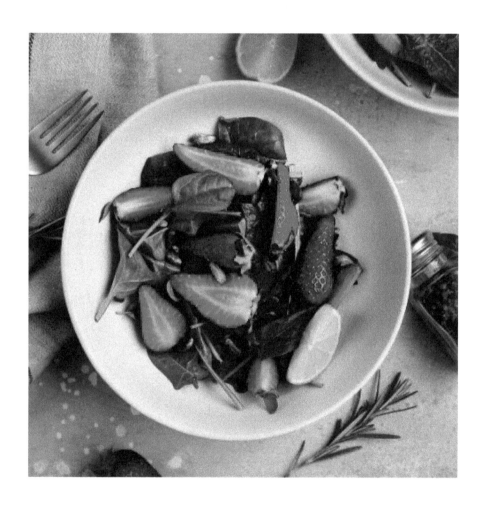

Spinach Berry Salad

🕐 Ready in about: 15 min.

🍴 Serves: 4

🍎 Per serving: Kcal 158, Sodium 198 mg, Protein 4 g, Carbs 25 g, Fat 5 g

INGREDIENTS

- 4 packed cups torn fresh spinach
- 1 cup sliced fresh strawberries
- 1 cup fresh or frozen blueberries
- 1 small, sweet onion, sliced
- ¼ cup chopped pecans, toasted
  Salad dressing:
- 2 tbsp. white wine vinegar or cider vinegar
- 2 tbsp. balsamic vinegar
- 2 tbsp. honey
- 2 tsp. Dijon mustard
- 1 tsp. curry powder (can be omitted)
- ⅛ tsp. pepper

DIRECTIONS

1. In a large bowl, combine the spinach, strawberries, blueberries, onion and pecans.

2. In a jar with a tight-fitting lid, combine the ingredients for the seasoning.

3. Shake well. Pour over salad and toss to coat.

4. Serve immediately.

DAY 5

BREAKFAST: Veggie Omelette

SNACK A.M.: 6 oz. blueberries

10 almonds

LUNCH: Chicken Fajitas

Snack P.M.: Fig Bars

DINNER: Black Bean Cakes & English Cucumber Salad

NUTRITIONAL VALUES:

Kcal: 1195

Sodium: 1041 mg

Protein: 62.5 g

Carbs: 87 g

Fat: 49 g

TO MAKE IT 1500 KCAL. ADD:

¼ cup unsalted dry-roasted almonds to breakfast
1 medium banana to lunch.

TO MAKE IT 2000 KCAL. ADD:

¼ cup unsalted dry-roasted almonds to breakfast
1 banana and a 1 oz. slice whole-wheat baguette to lunch
1 pear to P.M. snack

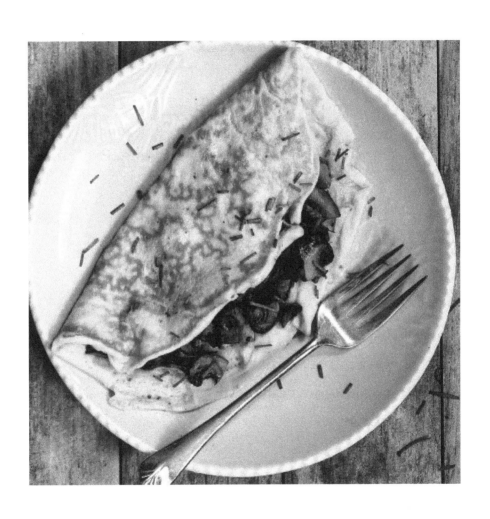

Veggie Omelette

🕐 **Ready in about: 15 min.**

🍴 **Serves: 1**

🍎 **Per serving: Kcal 279, Sodium 580 mg, Protein 22 g, Carbs 6 g, Fat 20 g**

INGREDIENTS

- 1 tbsp. extra virgin olive oil
- ¼ cup coarsely chopped broccoli
- 2 tbsp. chopped red onion
- 1 clove garlic, minced
- ¼ cup chopped zucchini
- 2 egg whites
- 1 whole egg
- ⅛ cup shredded low-fat cheddar cheese
- ⅛ tsp. sea salt
- ⅛ tsp. cracked black pepper

DIRECTIONS

1. Heat a medium non-stick skillet over medium heat and add the oil once the pan is hot.

2. When the oil is hot, add the broccoli and cook for a minute before adding the onion, garlic and zucchini.

3. Fry for 3-4 minutes. In a small bowl, beat the whites and the whole egg and season with salt and pepper.

4. Reduce the heat and add the beaten eggs to the pan with the vegetables, making sure to tilt the pan so that the eggs evenly coat the vegetables.

5. After 30 seconds, turn off the heat, turn the tortilla over and spread the cheese on half of the tortilla.

6. Overlay the other half over the cheese and cover the pan with a lid.

7. Cook, 1 to 2 minutes or until cheese is melted.

8. Serve immediately.

Chicken Fajitas

⏰ Ready in about: 20 min.

🍴 Serves: 4

🍎 Per serving: Kcal 453, Sodium 415 mg, Protein 32 g, Carbs 46 g, Fat 20.5 g

INGREDIENTS

Sauce

- ½ cup low-fat plain Greek yogurt
- 1 big avocado, pitted, peeled, and cut in fourths
- ¼ cup water
- ⅛ tsp. cracked black pepper
- ½ small serrano chile pepper
- Juice of ½ lemon
- ⅛ tsp. sea salt

Fajitas

- 4 (4 oz.) boneless, skinless chicken breasts, cut into ½-inch- thick strips
- ⅛ tsp. cracked black pepper
- ⅛ tsp. sea salt
- 2 large red bell peppers, cut into ½-inch-thick strips
- 1 tsp. dried oregano, divided
- 3 tbsp. extra virgin olive oil
- 2 large yellow bell peppers, cut into ½-inch- thick strips
- ¼ tsp. ground cumin
- 2 big green bell peppers, cut into ½-inch-thick strips
- 1 large white onion, cut into ½-inch slivers
- 2 large cloves garlic, minced
- 8 corn tortillas

DIRECTIONS

1. For the sauce, put all the ingredients in a blender and whisk until smooth. Set aside.
2. For the fajitas, season the chicken with salt, pepper, cumin, and half of the oregano.
3. Warmth the oil in a large saucepan over medium-high heat.
4. Once the oil is hot, add the chicken and cook for 4-5 minutes.
5. Add the peppers, onion, garlic, and remaining dried oregano.
6. Season with pepper and salt to taste and cook for a few more minutes, until the vegetables are soft.
7. Heat the tortillas in a skillet over low heat.
8. Pour the chicken and veggie mixture over each tortilla and drizzle with avocado sauce.
9. Fold the tortilla and serve.

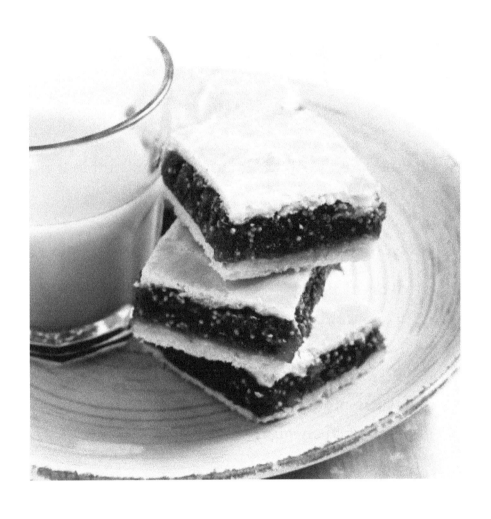

Fig Bars

⏰ **Ready in about: 45 min.**

🍴 **Serves: 36**

🍎 **Per serving: Kcal 92, Sodium 18 mg, Protein 2 g, Carbs 18 g, Fat 1.5 g**

INGREDIENTS

- **16 oz. dried figs**
- **½ cup walnuts**
- **1½ cups all-purpose flour**
- **½ tsp. baking soda**
- **1¼ cup old fashioned organic rolled oats**
- **1⅓ cup brown sugar**
- **½ cup butter**
- **4 cup orange juice**
- **2 tbsp. hot water**
- **cooking spray**

DIRECTIONS

1. Prepare an oven dish by spraying it with non-stick cooking spray.

2. Preheat the oven to 350°F.

3. In a mixing bowl, mix together the figs, orange juice, hot water, walnuts, and ⅓ cup sugar.

4. In another mixing bowl, mix together the 1 cup of sugar and butter until light and fluffy.

5. Add the egg to the sugar mixture and whisk it until it is smooth.

6. In an enormous mixing bowl, sift together the baking soda and flour.

7. Add the egg mixture to the flour and mix it into a soft dough.

8. Take one cup of the dough and put it aside. Press the rest of the dough into the bottom of the prepared baking tray.

9. Pour and spread the fig mixture evenly over the top of the pressed dough in the baking tray.

10. Crumble the remaining dough over the top of the fig mixture.

11. Place the fig mixture into the oven and bake for 25 to 30 minutes until the crust is golden brown.

12. When the fig bars are done, take them out of the oven and let them cool.

13. When the fig bar has cooled down, cut it into equal squares, and serve.

Black Bean Cakes

🕐 **Ready in about: 1 h 30 min.**

🍴 **Serves: 8**

🍎 **Per serving: Kcal 196, Sodium 156 mg, Protein 9.5 g, Carbs 31 g, Fat 7 g**

INGREDIENTS

- **2 tbsp. olive oil**
- **½ tsp. salt**
- **½ cup chopped fresh cilantro**
- **8 garlic cloves (chopped)**
- **2 cups water**
- **2 cups dried black beans (picked over, washed, soaked overnight, and drained)**

DIRECTIONS

1. Put water and black beans in a pan over high flame.
2. Bring to a boil.
3. Turn heat to low and simmer for 70 minutes while partially covered.
4. Drain the liquid.
5. Put garlic and beans in a bowl. Mash as you mix.
6. Add salt and cilantro. Mix well.
7. Use your hands to form 8 cakes from the mixture.
8. Arrange on a plate and keep in the fridge for an hour.
9. Heat up the oil in a pan over medium flame.
10. Cook the cakes for 5 minutes or until crisp.
11. Serve at once.

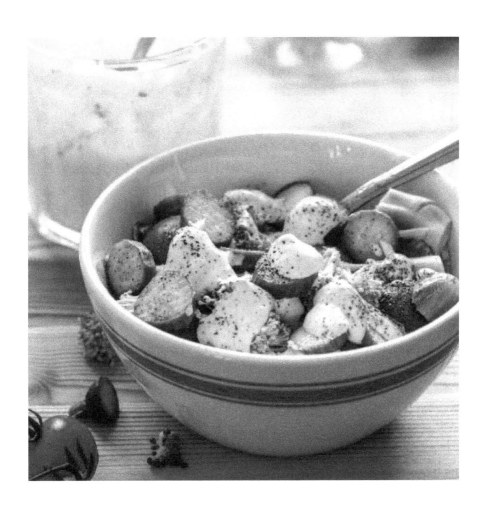

English Cucumber Salad

🕐 **Ready in about: 25 min.**

🍴 **Serves: 4**

🍎 **Per serving: Kcal 67, Sodium 90 mg, Protein 0.5 g, Carbs 5 g, Fat 5 g**

INGREDIENTS

- 1 English cucumber with peel (8 to 9 inches in length), washed and thinly sliced
- Cracked black pepper, to taste
  For the dressing:
- 1 tbsp. finely chopped fresh rosemary
- 2 tbsp. balsamic vinegar
- 1½ tbsp. olive oil
- 1 tbsp. low-salt Dijon mustard

DIRECTIONS

1. In a portable saucepan, add the vinegar, rosemary and olive oil.
2. Heat to mix and enhance the flavors over very low heat, approximately 5 minutes.
3. Take it out from the heat and add the mustard until well combined.
4. In a serving bowl, add the cucumber slices.
5. Pour the dressing over the cucumbers and toss to coat evenly.
6. Add black pepper to taste.
7. Refrigerate until ready to serve.

DAY 6

BREAKFAST: Apple and Cinnamon Oatmeal

SNACK A.M.: 4 oz. light yogurt, nonfat

1 oz. almonds

LUNCH: Rice and Beans Salad

Snack P.M.: ½ cup walnut halves

DINNER: Tomato Halibut Fillets

NUTRITIONAL VALUES:

 Kcal: 1150

Sodium: 455 mg

Protein: 90 g

Carbs: 109 g

Fat: 32 g

TO MAKE IT 1500 KCAL. ADD:

¼ cup unsalted dry-roasted almonds to breakfast

1 small apple to lunch

TO MAKE IT 2000 KCAL. ADD:

¼ cup unsalted dry-roasted almonds to breakfast

¼ cup walnuts to A.M. snack

1 medium apple to lunch

5 dried figs to P.M. snack

Apples and Cinnamon Oatmeal

⏰ **Ready in about: 20 min.**

🍴 **Serves: 2**

🍎 **Per serving: Kcal 377, Sodium 77 mg, Protein 13 g, Carbs 73 g, Fat 16 g**

INGREDIENTS

- 1½ cups unsweetened plain almond milk
- 1 cup old-fashioned oats
- 1 large, unpeeled Granny Smith apple, cubed
- ¼ tsp. ground cinnamon
- 2 tbsp. toasted walnut pieces

DIRECTIONS

1. Bring the milk to warmth over medium heat and add the oatmeal and apple.
2. Beat until almost all the liquid is absorbed, about 4 minutes.
3. Add the cinnamon.
4. Pour the oat mixture into two bowls and garnish with walnuts.

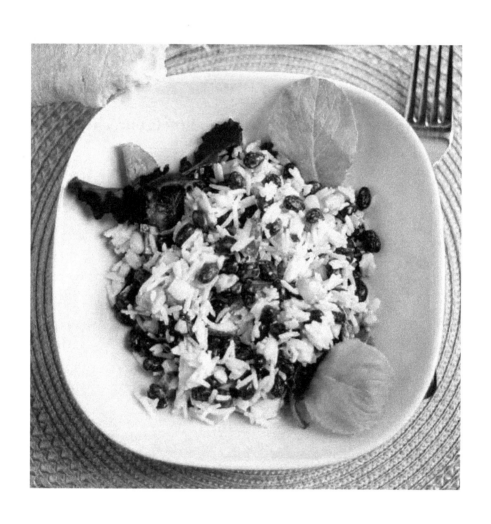

Rice and Beans Salad

🕐 **Ready in about: 3 h**

🍴 **Serves: 10**

🍎 **Per serving: Kcal 227, Sodium 110 mg, Protein 7 g, Carbs 34 g, Fat 7 g**

INGREDIENTS

- 1½ cups uncooked brown rice
- 3 cups of water
- ½ cup of chopped shallots or spring onions
- ½ cup chopped fresh parsley
- 15 oz. can unsalted garbanzo beans
- ¼ cup olive oil
- 15 oz. can unsalted dark kidney beans
- 1/3-½ cup rice vinegar, according to your taste

DIRECTIONS

1. Put the rice and water in the pot.
2. Cover and cook over medium heat until the rice is tender, about 45 to 50 minutes.
3. Let cool to room temperature.
4. Add the other ingredients.
5. Let cool for 2 hours or more.

Tomato Halibut Fillets

🕐 **Ready in about: 20 min.**

🍴 **Serves: 4**

🍎 **Per serving: Kcal 346, Sodium 158 mg, Protein 70 g, Carbs 2.5 g, Fat 9 g**

INGREDIENTS

- **2 tsp. sesame oil**
- **4 halibut fillets, skinless**
- **1 cup cherry tomatoes, halved**
- **1 tsp. dried basil**

DIRECTIONS

1. Sprinkle the fish with basil and place it in the hot pan.
2. Add the sesame oil and the cherry tomatoes.
3. Grill food for 4 minutes, then mix well and cook for another 5 minutes.
4. Serve hot.

DAY 7

BREAKFAST: Whole Grain Pancakes

SNACK A.M.: 1 medium apple

LUNCH: Mint Meatballs Spinach Sautè

Snack P.M.: 1 cup raspberries

DINNER: Baby Beet and Orange Salad & Salmon with Grated Beets

NUTRITIONAL VALUES:

Kcal: 1139

Sodium: 697 mg

Protein: 49 g

Carbs: 105 g

Fat: 35 g

TO MAKE IT 1500 KCAL. ADD:

¼ cup unsalted dry-roasted almonds to A.M. snack

½ cup cooked brown rice to dinner

TO MAKE IT 2000 KCAL. ADD:

1 slice whole-wheat toast with 1½ tbsp. almond butter and 1 small apple to breakfast

20 unsalted dry-roasted almonds to P.M. snack

½ cup cooked brown rice to dinner

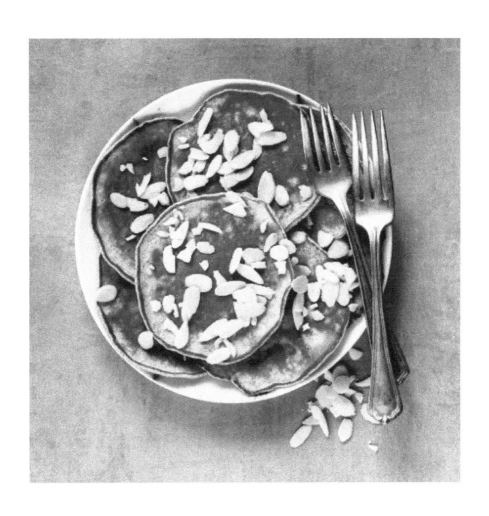

Whole Grain Pancakes

⏰ **Ready in about: 30 min.**

🍴 **Serves: 4**

🍎 **Per serving: Kcal 301, Sodium 483 mg, Protein 9 g, Carbs 55 g, Fat 10 g**

INGREDIENTS

- 1 tsp. vanilla extract
- 1 small banana, mashed
- 2 cups unsweetened almond milk
- ¼ cup unsweetened applesauce
- 1¼ cups whole wheat flour
- ¼ cup old-fashioned oats
- 2 tsp. baking powder
- ¼ tsp. sea salt
- ½ tsp. ground cinnamon
- 3 tbsp. brown sugar
- ½ cup of toasted almonds (chopped) or walnuts

DIRECTIONS

1. In a medium bowl, combine the wet ingredients.
2. In another larger bowl, combine the dry ingredients.
3. Add the wet ingredients to the dry ingredients and mix well until smooth.
4. Heat a roasting pan over medium heat, then coat with olive oil.
5. Use a ladle to pour the batter over the pan and cook the pancakes for 2-3 minutes.
6. Return them to a boil and continue cooking for about a minute.
7. Remove from heat and stack on a covered plate until all pancakes are cooked through.
8. Serve immediately.

Mint Meatballs Spinach Sautè

⏰ **Ready in about: 35 min.**

🍴 **Serves: 4**

🍎 **Per serving: Kcal 320, Sodium 250 mg, Protein 12 g, Carbs 16 g, Fat 13.5 g**

INGREDIENTS

- 1 yellow onion, chopped
- 1 pound pork stew meat, ground
- 1 egg, whisked
- Black pepper to the taste
- 1 tbsp. mint, chopped
- 2 garlic cloves, minced
- ½ cup low-sodium veggie stock
- 1 cup cherry tomatoes, halved
- 2 tbsp. olive oil

- 1 cup baby spinach

DIRECTIONS

1. In a portable bowl, combine the meat with the onion and the other ingredients except the oil, cherry tomatoes and the spinach, stir well and shape medium meatballs out of this mix.
2. Heat up a pan with the olive oil over medium-high heat, add the meatballs and cook them for 5 minutes on each side.
3. Add the spinach, tomatoes and the stock, toss, simmer everything for 15 minutes.
4. Divide everything into bowls and serve.

1.

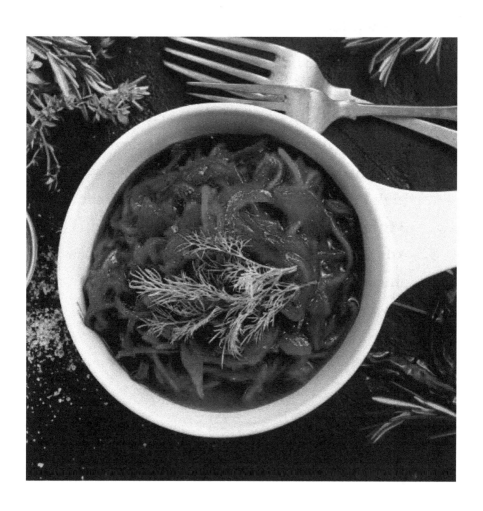

Baby Beet and Orange Salad

🕐 **Ready in about: 1h 25 min.**

🍴 **Serves: 4**

🍎 **Per serving: Kcal 118, Sodium 135 mg, Protein 3 g, Carbs 22 g, Fat 2 g**

INGREDIENTS

- 2 bunches baby beets with greens
- 2 ribs celery, chopped (½ cup)
- ¼ head Napa cabbage, chopped
- 1 chopped small yellow onion, chopped (½ cup)
- 1 orange, peeled and cut into segments
- Juice and zest of 1 orange
- ½ tbsp. olive oil
- black pepper to taste

DIRECTIONS

1. Warmth the oven to 400°F.
2. Cut the greens from the beets.
3. Rinse the greens under cold water, drain well and set aside.
4. Wash the beets. Pour a drizzle of olive oil on your hands and rub the beets to coat them lightly.
5. Wrap beets in foil and cook for about 45 minutes or until tender.
6. Allow it to cool until you can be able to handle it, then peel off the outer skin.
7. Cut and reserve. Cut the beets into strips and put them in the bowl.
8. Chop the celery, cabbage and onion and add them to the bowl.
9. Zest and juice one orange in the bowl.
10. Cut the already peeled orange into quarters.
11. Add to bowl. Pour half tbsp. of olive oil over the salad.
12. Top with black pepper and toss to combine.
13. Place the salad on cold plates and garnish with sliced beets.
14. Serve immediately.

Salmon with Grated Beets

⏰ **Ready in about: 20 min**

🍴 **Serves: 5**

🍎 **Per serving: Kcal 164, Sodium 75 mg, Protein 18.5 g, Carbs 2 g, Fat 9.5 g**

INGREDIENTS

- **2 oz. beetroot, grated**
- **½ tsp. minced garlic**
- **1 tsp. olive oil**
- **1-pound salmon fillet**
- **1 tbsp. mustard**
- **1 tbsp. margarine**

DIRECTIONS

1. Spread the salmon with the mustard and put it in the pan.

2. Add the margarine and grill the fish for 4 minutes on each side.

3. Meanwhile, add the minced garlic, grated beetroot and olive oil.

4. Garnish the cooked salmon fillets with beetroot.

passo pas paso mm	int. núcleo φ mm	broca φ mm
	2.46	2.5
0.5	3.24	3.3
0.7	4.13	4.
0.8	4.92	
1	6.65	
1.25	8.38	

APPENDIX WITH CONVERSION CHARTS

WEIGHTS	
IMPERIAL	**METRIC**
½ oz.	15 g
¾ oz.	20 g
1 oz.	30 g
2 oz.	60 g
3 oz.	85 g
16 oz. = 1 pound= 435 g	
1 oz. = 28.35 g | 1 g = 0.035 oz.	

LIQUIDS

CUPS	METRIC	PINT	QUART
1/4	60 ml	-	-
1/2	125 ml	-	-
-	150 ml	1/4	-
-	200 ml	-	-
1	250 ml	1/2	-
-	300 ml	-	-
-	400 ml	-	-
2	500 ml	-	-
-	950 ml	-	1

SPOONS

LIQUID		DRY	
¼ tsp.	1.25 ml	¼ tsp.	1.1 g
½ tsp.	2.5 ml	½ tsp.	2.3 g
1 tsp.	5 ml	1 tsp.	4.7 g
¼ tbsp.	3.75 ml	¼ tbsp.	3.5 g
½ tbsp.	7.5 ml	½ tbsp.	7.1 g
1 tbsp.	15 ml	1 tbsp.	14.3 g

OVEN TEMPS

°F	°C
250	120
275	140
300	150
325	170
350	180
375	190
400	200

COMMON INGREDIENTS

1 CUP	IMPERIAL	METRIC
Flour	5 oz.	140 g
Almonds	4 oz.	110 g
Uncooked Rice	6½ oz.	190 g
Brown Sugar	6½ oz.	185 g
Raisins	7 oz.	200 g
Grated Cheese	4 oz.	115 g

NOTES

CPSIA information can be obtained
at www.ICGtesting.com
Printed in the USA
LVHW080517250321
682338LV00014B/519